The 4-minute Neurologic Exam

(An answer to the "Neuro WNL" problem)

STEPHEN GOLDBERG, M.D.

Associate Professor
Department of Family Medicine
Department of Anatomy and Cell Biology
University of Miami School of Medicine

ISBN # 0-940780-05-4

Made in the United States of America

Published by
MedMaster, Inc.
P.O. Box 640028
Miami, FL 33164

TO MORTON E. FREIMAN, M.D., an angel in disguise

Contents

Preface

"NEURO WNL" ("the neurological exam is within normal limits") is commonly the last notation on a physical exam report. Regretfully, this often means that virtually no neuro exam took place. The patient looked O.K. to all superficial appearances and had no particular neurologic complaints. A physician can be trapped into this approach, when there is inadequate time for the 90 minute neurologic exam some references suggest, or even the 20 minute exam suggested for patients with no neurologic complaints. In reality, there are times when 5 minutes or less is available. This book, written for the non-neurologist, focuses on a brief neurologic screening exam that maximizes the useful information obtainable *when time is limited*. It is not a substitute for the more formal neurologic evaluation that should follow, perhaps by a neurologist, when the screening exam reveals significant findings.

A glossary has been included for words not defined in the text. Chapter 1 has been modified from an article by the author in the April 1981 issue of *American Family Physician*, and contains illustrations by Peter Y. Stone. Other illustrations are by the author. I thank Dr. Joseph Berger for his helpful comments and Ms. Beryn Frank for editing the manuscript. The cover illustration is a wood Marquetry reconstruction by John N. Beck of Sir Luke Fields' painting "The Doctor".

Chapter 1

PRINCIPLES OF NEUROLOGIC LOCALIZATION

The first step in neurologic evaluation is to determine that there is a neurologic problem and to localize the site of the lesion. Next, one must determine the cause of the lesion (hemorrhage, tumor, infections, etc.). The final step is to decide how to resolve the problem (surgery, medical treatment, etc.). Clinically relevant anatomic points in neuroanatomy, summarized in this chapter, are important in localizing a lesion.

Problems of neuroanatomical localization commonly present as radicular pain, numbness, tingling, visual disturbances, hearing deficits, dizziness, weakness, tremors and incoordination. The primary care physician need not locate a lesion causing neurologic symptoms *very precisely*. Whether the patient has an organic problem and whether the lesion is localized to the peripheral nerves, spinal cord, brainstem or higher centers *is* important.

ORGANIC OR NONORGANIC?

Malingering involves a willful faking of symptoms. In contrast, hysterical symptoms are psychogenic in nature, real to the patient's conscious mind, even though the neurologic examination may not make sense physiologically. The paraplegic patient who walks when no one is looking can be labeled a malingerer. Litigation often suggests, but certainly does not prove, malingering. Frequently malingering is difficult to distinguish from hysteria, and usually it is best to simply label the condition as "nonorganic", or "nonphysiologic".

Nonorganic symptoms can sometimes be identified by neuroanatomy. For instance, a patient may describe right-sided headaches, as well as loss of hearing, sight, smell, taste, sensation and motor ability on the right side. The problem is nonorganic in origin because it requires multiple lesions, all coincidentally resulting in right-sided symptoms. The condition does not make sense neuroanatomically. Nonorganic signs also include the following:

1. The hand of a patient in feigned coma released from above his head will not strike his face, because the patient does not want to hurt himself.

2. Nonorganic total blindness is unmasked by the demonstration of eye movements that follow a moving object.

3. The patient with 20/200 vision at 20 feet has a nonorganic problem if he reads no better than the same 20/200 line at 2 feet.

4. Diplopia, except in rare instances (dislocated lens, retinal detachment) should disappear when one eye is covered.

5. In nonorganic anosmia, the patient fails to react to ammonia. In true anosmia, it should be sensed because ammonia acts by stimulating the pain endings of the trigeminal nerve.

6. It is nonorganic for a patient to report absent position sense upon ankle dorsiflexion but then walk with the eyes closed, an act that depends on this sensory input.

7. A nonorganic condition is apparent in the patient who exhibits a reflex before the tendon is tapped.

8. It is not physiologic for a patient to complain of joint weakness and simultaneously contract the joint extensors and flexors when asked to move the joint. (In flexion, the extensors normally relax and vice versa).

9. Discrepancies in pain when assuming a jackknife position may also indicate a nonorganic problem—for instance, a supine patient who reports back pain on lifting the legs to the trunk but has no significant pain from the same maneuver while sitting.

Organic disease is suggested by signs that cannot be faked: significant asymmetry in the pupillary light reflex, abnormal retinal appearance, ocular divergence, marked nystagmus, muscle atrophy and fasciculation. Multiple complex signs and symptoms that can be explained by a single small lesion also suggest organic disease.

The detection of nonorganic signs does not necessarily mean that the patient's entire condition is nonorganic. A patient may have an organic problem with an hysterical overlay. In complex cases, referral to a neurologist may be necessary to avoid excessive invasive testing or inadvertent dismissal of a potentially serious organic problem.

NEUROANATOMY

Figure 1 is a schematic outline of the major motor and sensory pathways. A lesion of the pain-temperature pathway (spinothalamic tract), whether within the brain stem or spinal cord, will result in loss of pain-temperature sensation contralaterally, below the level of the lesion.

A lesion at the spinal level of the pathway for conscious proprioception (the ability to sense the position and movement of the limbs) and stereognosis (the ability to identify objects by touch) will result in loss of these senses ipsilaterally, below the level of the lesion.

The path for light touch combines features of these two pathways. Consequently, light touch typically is spared in unilateral spinal cord lesions because there are alternate routes to carry the information.

All of these sensory pathways eventually cross the midline, synapse in the thalamus and terminate in the sensory area of the cerebrum. Therefore, a lesion of the sensory area of the cerebral

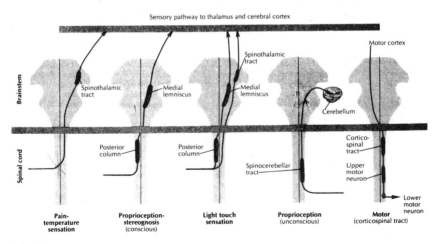

Fig. 1

cortex results in contralateral deficits in pain-temperature, proprioception, stereognosis and light touch sensation.

Proprioception has a conscious and an unconscious component. The conscious pathway connects with the thalamus and cerebral cortex, enabling one to describe the position of a limb. The unconscious pathway (spinocerebellar tract) connects with the cerebellum, which is considered an unconscious organ, and enables one to walk and perform other complex acts without having to think about which joints to flex and extend. Unlike the other sensory pathways, which cross contralaterally, the spinocerebellar tract primarily remains ipsilateral. In general, one side of the cerebellum influences the same side of the body. Thus cerebellar lesions tend to produce ipsilateral malfunction, typically presenting as ataxia (awkwardness of movement), whereas cerebral lesions result in contralateral defects, manifested by weakness or sensory loss.

The corticospinal tract and related motor pathways (not shown in figure 1) synapse in the spinal cord, just before leaving the cord. This anatomic feature is important because motor neurons above the level of this synapse are *upper motor neurons (UMN),* and the peripheral nerve cell bodies and their extensions beyond this synapse are *lower motor neurons (LMN).* Upper and lower motor neuron injuries produce different clinical signs. Although a disorder at either level results in weakness, the presentations differ (Fig. 2).

CEREBRAL LESIONS

An unilateral cerebral cortex lesion commonly results in weakness and sensory loss in the contralateral extremities. However, unilateral cerebral cortex lesions do not affect all cranial nerves,

---

Clinical Findings in Upper and Lower Motor Neuron Defects

Upper motor neuron defect

Spastic weakness
No significant muscle atrophy
No fasciculations and fibrillations
Hyperreflexia
Babinski reflex may be present

Lower motor neuron defect

Flaccid weakness
Significant atrophy
Fasciculations and fibrillations
Hyporeflexia
No Babinski reflex

Fig. 2

because of bilateral representation of function: one side of the cerebrum, rather than connecting entirely with the cranial nerves on the opposite side of the body, connects with most cranial nerves on both sides of the body. Therefore, a lesion to one side of the cerebrum will cause little, if any, deficit in certain cranial nerve functions, as connections from the other side of the cerebrum maintain function. For example, hoarseness may represent a lesion of the 10th cranial nerve but will not stem from a unilateral cerebral cortex lesion.

Cerebral lesions affect the cranial nerves as follows:

Olfactory Nerve (CN1). This nerve does not cross the midline; consequently, a unilateral cortical lesion results in ipsilateral anosmia.

Optic (CN2), Oculomotor (CN3), Trochlear (CN4) and Abducens (CN6) Nerves. Destruction of a cerebral hemisphere does not result in visual loss or ocular paralysis that is confined to the contralateral eye. Rather, both eyes are partially affected. Regarding motor function, neither eye can move to the contralateral side (the eyes "look toward the lesion"). Regarding sensory function, neither eye sees the contralateral environment. Figure 3 illustrates how a lesion of the left optic tract results in loss of the right visual field in each eye.

The pupillary light reflex is consensual; that is, light information from one eye is relayed to the brainstem via CN2 and back to both eyes via CN3 on each side, causing both pupils to constrict. This is a brainstem-mediated reflex; cerebral lesions do not eliminate it. Figure 4 summarizes the changes in the pupillary light reflex following CN2 or CN3 injury.

Trigeminal Nerve (CN5). A cerebral lesion results in loss of sensation on the opposite side of the face.

Facial Nerve (CN7). Cerebral lesions generally only result in paralysis of the lower half of the face (below the eye) contralaterally, due to the bilateral connections to the forehead and eyelids from each hemisphere. When the facial nerve itself is damaged, as in Bell's palsy, there is total ipsilateral hemifacial paralysis, including the forehead and the eyelids; the patient cannot raise the eyebrow or close the eyelids on one side.

Vestibulocochlear Nerve (CN8). Hearing deficits result from local lesions between the ear and the brainstem. A lesion in one hemisphere results in little deficit, because auditory information from

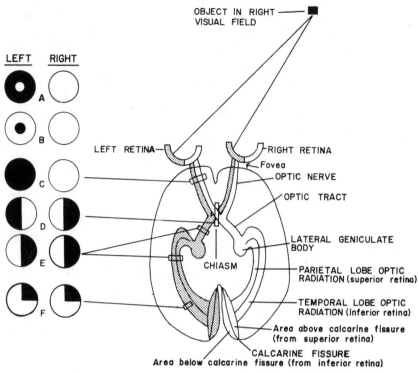

Fig. 3   The visual pathways as seen from above the brain. Letters A–F refer to visual field defects following lesions in the corresponding brain areas. Circles indicate what the left and right eyes see (the left and right visual fields). Black areas represent visual field defects. A. Constricted field left eye (e.g., end-stage glaucoma). When constricted fields are bilateral, it sometimes signifies hysteria. B. Central scotoma (e.g., optic neuritis in multiple sclerosis). C. Total blindness of the left eye. D. Bitemporal hemianopia (e.g., pituitary gland tumor). E. Right homonymous hemianopia (e.g. stroke). F. Right superior quandrantopia.

Pupillary Reaction Following Total Optic or Oculomotor Nerve Injury

Injury	Light shined in right eye	Light shined in left eye
Right optic nerve (CN 2)	No response in either pupil	Both pupils constrict
Right oculomotor nerve (CN 3)	Only left pupil constricts	Only left pupil constricts

Fig. 4

each ear is represented bilaterally. Auditory fibers, upon entering the brainstem, immediately divide into ipsilateral and contralateral routes that go to both cerebral hemispheres.

Vertigo suggests a deficit in the peripheral vestibular apparatus, vestibular nerve or brainstem (rarely the cortex). A brainstem etiology becomes more suspect when there are accompanying brain stem signs that suggest involvement of long sensory or motor pathways which pass through the brainstem and spinal cord.

Glossopharyngeal (CN9), Vagus (CN10), Accessory (CN11) and Hypoglossal (CN12) Nerves. Except for CN12, these nerves are not significantly affected by unilateral cerebral lesions. Weakness of one-half of the tongue may occur sometimes with a contralateral cerebral lesion, but is more striking with a direct lesion of CN12.

PERIPHERAL NERVE OR CENTRAL NERVOUS SYSTEM LESION?

A sensory deficit along a dermatome, particularly when accompanied by local pain, suggests a peripheral nerve lesion (Fig. 5). The peripheral nervous system is neatly partitioned along dermatomes, whereas the central nervous system is not. Lesions of sensory tracts within the CNS characteristically present as general defects in an extremity rather than specific dermatome deficits. In addition, CNS lesions involve loss of sensation rather than cause pain. An exception is the rare thalamic pain syndrome, in which a thalamic lesion may produce vague, difficult-to localize pain. Lower or upper motor neuron signs may be used to further distinguish peripheral and CNS lesions (Fig. 2).

Figures 6 and 7 illustrate the motor and sensory deficits that arise from classic peripheral nerve lesions. Deficits due to lesions of spinal nerve roots, peripheral nerve plexuses and more peripheral extensions of the nerve differ in complex ways, because peripheral plexuses and nerves are mixtures of fibers arising from several nerve roots.

SPINAL CORD, BRAINSTEM INTERNAL CAPSULE OR CEREBRAL LESION?

The combination of UMN signs with a spinal dermatome defect suggests a CNS lesion involving the spinal nerve roots, specifically a spinal cord problem. In addition, dissociation of sensory mod-

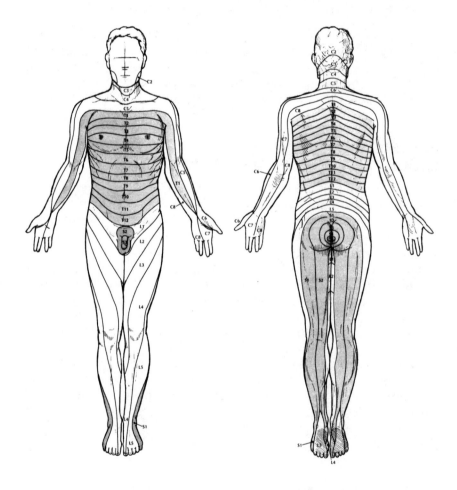

Peripheral Nerve Injuries and Their Associated Motor Deficits

Nerve	Motor functions impaired with injury
Radial (C5-C8)	Elbow and wrist extension (patient has wrist drop); extension of fingers at metacarpophalangeal joints; triceps reflex
Median (C6-T1)	Wrist, thumb, index and middle finger flexion; thumb opposition, forearm pronation; ability of wrist to bend toward the radial (thumb) side; atrophy of thenar eminence (ball of thumb)
Ulnar (C8-T1)	Flexion of wrist, ring and small fingers (claw hand); opposition of little finger; ability of wrist to bend toward ulnar (small finger) side; adduction and abduction of fingers; atrophy of hypothenar eminence of the palm (at base of ring and small fingers)
Musculocutaneous (C5-C6)	Elbow flexion (biceps); forearm supination; biceps reflex
Axillary (C5-C6)	Ability to move upper arm outward, forward or backward (deltoid atrophy)
Long thoracic (C5-C7)	Ability to elevate arm above horizontal (patient has winging of scapula)
Femoral (L2-L4)	Knee extension; hip flexion; knee jerk
Obturator (L2-L4)	Hip adduction (patient's leg swings outward when walking)
Sciatic (L4-S3)	Knee flexion plus other functions along its branches (tibial and common peroneal nerves)
Tibial (L4-S3)	Foot inversion; ankle plantar flexion; ankle jerk
Common peroneal (L4-S2)	Foot eversion; ankle and toes dorsiflexion (patient has high slapping gait due to foot drop). This nerve is *commonly* injured.

Fig. 6

alities suggests a spinal cord lesion: e.g., loss of pain-temperature sensation in the right leg and loss of proprioception in the left leg. Only at the spinal cord level can a single lesion produce this deficit. The sensory modalities from a given body region are separated on either side of the spinal cord. Above the level of the spinal cord, the pathways for the various sensory modalities are situated on the same side of the brainstem and brain (Fig. 1).

Cranial nerve dysfunction indicates a lesion above the foramen magnum. If a cranial nerve deficit is on one side, combined with a contralateral extremity hemiparesis or hemianesthesia (e.g., right facial paralysis and left hemiplegia), the patient must have a brainstem lesion. In such a case, a cerebral cortex lesion can be ruled out because it would present with a deficit confined to the contralateral side (e.g. left facial paralysis and left hemiplegia).

A cranial nerve or brainstem lesion, rather than a cerebral cortex lesion, is suggested in any of the following kinds of cranial nerve involvement: loss of vision in one eye (CN2), pupillary inequality or difficulty in moving one eye (CN3,4, or 6), marked unilateral weakness of the masseter muscle (CN5), total unilateral facial

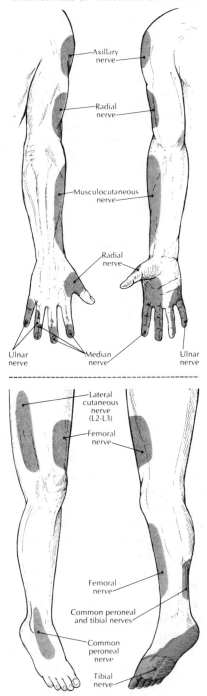

Fig. 7. Sensory defects following peripheral nerve injuries.

paralysis (CN7), unilateral hearing loss (CN8), difficulty in swallowing (CN9 and/or 10), hoarseness (CN10) or difficulty in raising the shoulder or turning the head (CN11). The bilateral connections of the cerebral cortex to the cranial nerves obviate the possibility of such cranial nerve signs in unilateral cerebral lesions.

Bilateral lesions of the cerebral cortex or internal capsule (the area where cerebral cortex fibers funnel into the brainstem) may results in *pseudobulbar palsy*, in which there are multiple cranial nerve deficits. The patient experiences difficulties with facial expression, movement of the tongue, chewing, swallowing, speech and breathing. There also may be inappropriate spells of laughing or crying.

It may be difficult to differentiate a lesion in the cerebral cortex from one in the internal capsule. The presence of a higher level dysfunction suggests a cerebral cortex lesion. This may include an agnosia (complex receptive disability, e.g., loss of ability to understand what one is reading while retaining the ability to see), apraxia (complex motor disability, such as putting on one's pants backwards), and aphasia (complex speech disturbance, as opposed to simple hoarseness or monotone).

CEREBELLAR OR BASAL GANGLIA LESION?

Awkwardness of movement, as opposed to weakness, is characteristic of both cerebellar and basal ganglia lesions. Awkwardness of *intended* movements (e.g. intention tremor, ataxia) suggests a lesion of the cerebellum or its connecting pathways. *Involuntary* movements (e.g., resting tremor, chorea, athetosis, hemiballismus) are characteristic of basal ganglia lesions.

REVIEW: Figure 8 shows 24 classic problems of neurologic localization. The shaded areas indicate regions of functional deficit.

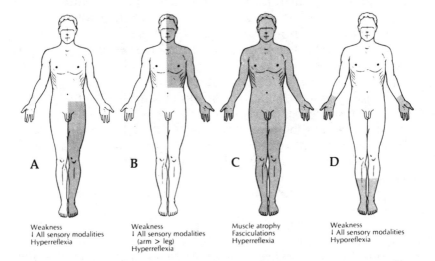

A

Weakness
↓ All sensory modalities
Hyperreflexia

B

Weakness
↓ All sensory modalities
  (arm > leg)
Hyperreflexia

C

Muscle atrophy
Fasciculations
Hyperreflexia

D

Weakness
↓ All sensory modalities
Hyporeflexia

Fig. 8. A. Right anterior cerebral artery occlusion. The anterior cerebral artery predominantly supplies the area of the cerebral cortex that controls the opposite lower extremity. The leg is generally most affected.

B. Right middle cerebral artery occlusion. The middle cerebral artery predominantly supplies the area of the cerebral cortex that controls the opposite upper half of the body. The proximal lower extremity is also commonly involved.

C. Amyotrophic lateral sclerosis. The combination of upper and lower motor neuron signs is diagnostic. Distal extremities commonly are affected first.

D. Peripheral neuropathy. It may present in a dermatome distribution or, as in the depiction, in a glove-and-stocking distribution. Nonorganic sensory disorders also commonly present in a glove-and-stocking distribution.

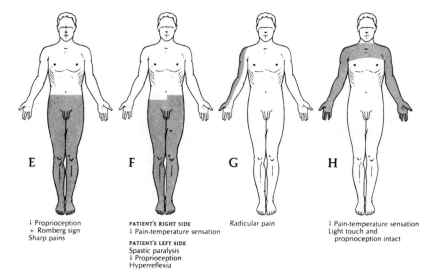

E
| Proprioception
+ Romberg sign
Sharp pains

F
PATIENT'S RIGHT SIDE
| Pain-temperature sensation

PATIENT'S LEFT SIDE
Spastic paralysis
| Proprioception
Hyperreflexia

G
Radicular pain

H
| Pain-temperature sensation
Light touch and
proprioception intact

Fig. 8. E. Neurosyphilis (tabes dorsalis). Posterior columns are characteristically affected, leading to Romberg's sign (the patient falls on closing the eyes, due to the loss of proprioception). Upper extremities are less commonly affected.

F. Hemisection of the spinal cord on the left, at T11 (Brown-Séquard syndrome). Note the sensory dissociation.

G. Radicular pain, cervical roots C5-C6.

H. Syringomyelia. Pain-temperature fibers that cross the spinal cord midline are affected. Cervical levels are most commonly affected. Often, there is atrophy of the small muscles of the hand when the lesion extends from the midline to the adjacent motor horn cells.

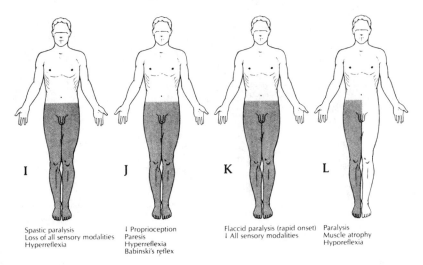

I   J

Spastic paralysis   ↓ Proprioception
Loss of all sensory modalities   Paresis
Hyperreflexia   Hyperreflexia
                                   Babinski's reflex

K   L

Flaccid paralysis (rapid onset)   Paralysis
↓ All sensory modalities   Muscle atrophy
                                   Hyporeflexia

Fig. 8. I. Total transection of the spinal cord at T11. A lesion of the cerebral midline is a possible alternative diagnosis but the signs would probably be less severe and less sharply defined than those following spinal cord transection.

J. Pernicious anemia. Proprioceptive and corticospinal pathways are characteristically affected. Commonly, there is also numbness and tingling of the distal portion of all extremities, secondary to peripheral nerve involvement.

K. Guillain-Barré syndrome. Peripheral nerve roots are affected. Polyneuritis commonly ascends to the upper extremities and face after affecting the lower extremities. The motor deficit tends to be more prominent than the sensory deficit.

L. Poliomyelitis. Motor horn cell bodies of peripheral nerves are affected, leading to lower motor neuron signs.

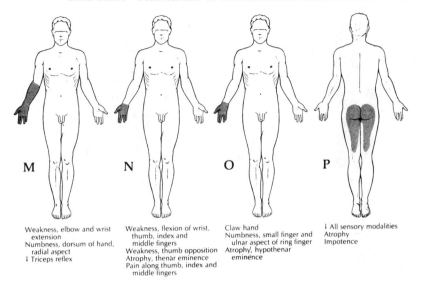

Weakness, elbow and wrist extension	Weakness, flexion of wrist, thumb, index and middle fingers	Claw hand	↓ All sensory modalities

M: Weakness, elbow and wrist extension / Numbness, dorsum of hand, radial aspect / ↓ Triceps reflex

N: Weakness, flexion of wrist, thumb, index and middle fingers / Weakness, thumb opposition / Atrophy, thenar eminence / Pain along thumb, index and middle fingers

O: Claw hand / Numbness, small finger and ulnar aspect of ring finger / Atrophy, hypothenar eminence

P: ↓ All sensory modalities / Atrophy / Impotence

Fig. 8. M. Radial nerve injury.

N. Proximal median nerve injury. If the lesion were distal at the level of the wrist (carpal tunnel syndrome), wrist flexion would not be affected.

O. Ulnar nerve injury.

P. Cauda equina lesion, S2-S4.

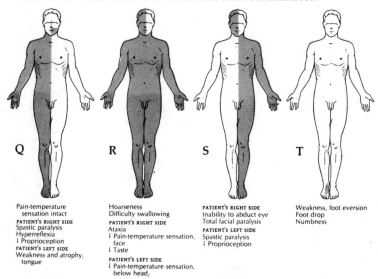

Q

Pain-temperature
  sensation intact
PATIENT'S RIGHT SIDE
Spastic paralysis
Hyperreflexia
↓ Proprioception
PATIENT'S LEFT SIDE
Weakness and atrophy,
  tongue

R

Hoarseness
Difficulty swallowing
PATIENT'S RIGHT SIDE
Ataxia
↓ Pain-temperature sensation,
  face
↓ Taste
PATIENT'S LEFT SIDE
↓ Pain-temperature sensation,
  below head

S

PATIENT'S RIGHT SIDE
Inability to abduct eye
Total facial paralysis
PATIENT'S LEFT SIDE
Spastic paralysis
↓ Proprioception

T

Weakness, foot eversion
Foot drop
Numbness

Fig. 8. Q. R and S. Brainstem lesions. Note the combination of cranial nerve deficits and contralateral extremity defects.

Q and R depict lesions involving the medulla. Sensation on the most medial aspect of the face may be spared with medullary lesions.

S represents a lesion of the pons.

T. Common peroneal nerve injury.

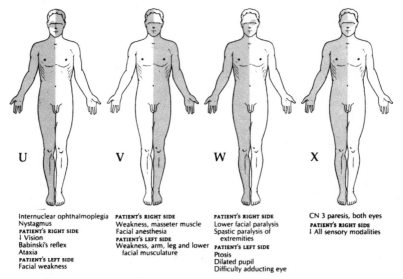

U	V	W	X
Internuclear ophthalmoplegia	**PATIENT'S RIGHT SIDE**	**PATIENT'S RIGHT SIDE**	CN 3 paresis, both eyes
Nystagmus	Weakness, masseter muscle	Lower facial paralysis	**PATIENT'S RIGHT SIDE**
PATIENT'S RIGHT SIDE	Facial anesthesia	Spastic paralysis of	↓ All sensory modalities
↓ Vision	**PATIENT'S LEFT SIDE**	extremities	
Babinski's reflex	Weakness, arm, leg and lower	**PATIENT'S LEFT SIDE**	
Ataxia	facial musculature	Ptosis	
PATIENT'S LEFT SIDE		Dilated pupil	
Facial weakness		Difficulty adducting eye	

Fig. 8. U. Multiple sclerosis. No single lesion possible.

V, W and X. Brainstem lesions. Cranial nerve defects are present on one side, with involvement of the extremities on the opposite side.

V indicates a lesion of the pons.

W and X illustrate a lesion of the midbrain.

Chapter 2

HISTORY

As in other areas of medicine, the history component of the neurologic examination frequently provides more useful information than the physical exam or laboratory tests. This section discusses key diagnostic questions in the evaluation of the most common symptoms and signs.

The neurologic history follows the same overall format as any general medical history. After eliciting the chief complaint, the history of the present illness must be taken with great care.

History of Present Illness

Understand the main complaint.

A. What is it that the patient is feeling?
B. When did the problem begin and how did it progress?
C. Is there anything that makes it feel better or worse?
D. Are there any other associated symptoms?

HEADACHE

What type of pain is the patient feeling? It is constant or throbbing? Throbbing is more suggestive of a *vascular* cause. Intermittent lightning-like jabs over the trigeminal nerve distribution are characteristic of *trigeminal neuralgia*. Where is the headache located? *Migraine* headaches commonly show a predilection for one side of the head but should occur on the opposite side at least occasionally. If a headache always occurs only on the same side, suspect an underlying lesion, which will constantly refer pain to the same side of the head. *Sinus headaches* refer to the respective sinuses and are painful on direct pressure. The headaches of acute angle closure *glaucoma* and *uveitis* center around the eye and are associated with a red eye and visual loss. *Tension headaches* commonly refer to the top of the head, the neck, or to a band-like area around the temples, and may include the eyes. The headache in *meningitis* and *subarachnoid* hemorrhage is likely to localize to the back of the neck; it is associated with neck stiffness during neck flexion, and often with pain spreading down the back.

How did the headache progress? A headache that has been intermittent over many years is less ominous than one that just recently occurred (particularly in an elderly person). The headache of *subarachnoid hemorrhage* characteristically occurs suddenly, whereas those of tumors generally progress over weeks or months.

Does anything make the headache feel better or worse? How does it feel to press on the site of pain? Infections or inflammations (as in *sinusitis* or *temporal arteritis*) usually feel worse on direct pressure. Tension and migraine headaches usually do not feel worse on direct pressure and often may feel better. Is it worse in the day or at night? *Cluster headaches* are severe unilateral headaches that occur particularly at night and often are worse with alcohol ingestion (they are also associated with a red eye). They commonly are "clustered", with remissions and exacerbations occurring over weeks or months. Headaches resulting from *intracranial lesions* may also occur at night. Trigeminal neuralgia attacks commonly are precipitated by chewing or touching a particular area of the face, such as the nose or mouth.

Are there any other associated symptoms? It is uncommon for headache to be the only initial manifestation of a brain tumor. As the brain has no pain endings, generally a tumor will first present with other neurologic findings (e.g., altered mental state, weakness, sensory loss, incoordination) before becoming large enough to affect pain endings in brain-contiguous structures, as the meninges. Suspect an extracranial source if pain is the only manifestation; the vast majority of headaches have an extracranial origin. Do any other symptoms immediately precede the headache? In classic migraine, there is a preceding *aura*, commonly a visual disturbance in one or both eyes (e.g., a wavy distortion, or scotoma, in front of one or both eyes, dizziness, nausea, and sometimes hemisensory or motor deficits).

DIZZINESS

What does the patient mean by "dizzy"? Vertigo (a sense of spinning of the person or environment) suggests a lesion of the vestibular apparatus, vestibular nerve, or junction of vestibular nerve with the brain stem. "Lightheadedness" or "faintness" suggest impairment of brain oxygenation, as by cardiac arrhythmia, or hypotension, or psychological factors.

Is the feeling worse on standing or lying down or during any particular activity? Orthostatic hypotension improves on lying down. The vertigo of subclavian steal worsens on movement of the affected upper limb.

Are there other associated symptoms? Coinciding palpitations, angina, or shortness of breath should raise the question of a cardiac cause of dizziness.

VISUAL DISTURBANCE

What is the patient experiencing? Does the visual disturbance affect one or both eyes? Monocular visual loss indicates a problem anterior to the optic chiasm. Binocular problems originate at, or posterior to, the optic chiasm unless there are separate lesions of the optic nerves or retinae. Figure 3 indicates the characteristic field defects in various conditions. Is the loss constant or intermittent? Intermittent, brief visual loss is characteristic of *transient ischemic attacks* as may occur with emboli or migraine. In *migraine* the field often has a wavy appearance. In *retinal detachment* there is the feeling of a curtain being drawn over a particular sector of the eye, and it does not improve of its own accord. In *acute (angle closure) glaucoma*, the patient may see rainbows or halos on viewing lights. With *digitalis toxicity* the visual field may have a yellowish hue. With central scotomata, the patient has profound difficulty with reading, but otherwise can navigate fairly well because peripheral vision is intact. With peripheral field losses, the patient may read excellently but bumps into objects because side vision is defective.

How did the problem begin and progress? Acute visual loss suggests a vascular origin. Retinal detachment may progress over minutes or hours. Tumors may progress over months. Retinal degenerations may progress over years. Multiple sclerosis may be marked by remissions and exacerbations of visual loss over periods of weeks, months, or years.

Does anything make the vision better or worse? If the problem is improved by glasses or by reading at a particular distance, this indicates a refractive error.

Are there other associated symptoms? In migraine, the visual disturbance commonly precedes a throbbing headache and/or other neurologic signs, like dizziness, nausea, weakness, or sensory loss. In uveitis and acute angle closure glaucoma, there may be intense pain about a red eye. In central nervous system lesions, there may be other neurologic signs suggesting the involvement of areas that border the visual pathways.

TREMOR

Is it the fine tremor that often is seen with anxiety or in benign familial conditions? Or is it a coarse 4–6 cycle/second "pill-rolling" tremor that is commonly seen in Parkinson's disease?

Is the tremor worse when the limb is at rest or when doing something? Parkinsonian tremor characteristically is worse at rest. Essential (benign, familial) tremor and tremors of cerebellar disease are worse on intention. Parkinsonian tremor (and that of anxiety) worsens on excitement and disappears during sleep.

Are there any other associated symptoms? In Parkinson's disease, stiffness and slowness of movements frequently accompany the tremor.

WEAKNESS AND SENSORY LOSS

Does the patient mean weakness in the paretic sense or is it a mental sense of "tiredness"? Is it "slowness", as in Parkinson's disease or myotonia? In *Parkinson's disease* the strength may be normal, but the patient takes a long time to act. In *myotonia*, there may be slowness in *release* of a hand grasp. In *myasthenia gravis*, there may be initial good strength, developing into marked paresis on successive repetitions of the same act. Does the patient complaining of "weakness" mean "pain" that decreases mobility, as in arthritis or bursitis?

For *sensory loss*, when the patient says "numb", does this mean loss of feeling, or weakness? Patients sometimes use the term "numb" when describing weakness. For "pain", "burning", "tingling", is it deep or superficial, the latter suggesting an involvement of cutaneous nerves as in *herpes zoster, peripheral neuropathy*, and other nerve dysfunctions. Deep pain should call to mind additional potential factors—trauma, arthritis, inflammations, infections, or tumors.

How did it progress? Strokes characteristically arise suddenly or are rapidly progressive over hours, then stabilizing. Transient ischemic attacks occur suddenly but then improve over a few minutes or hours. *Todd's paralysis* immediately following an epileptic seizure disappears within a few hours or days (there may also be transient sensory disturbances, visual defects, and aphasia). Tumors gradually progress and do not improve, with uncommon exceptions. Multiple sclerosis comes and goes intermittently over periods of weeks, months, or years. Symptoms of subdural hematomas may arise suddenly or progress over weeks if there is gradual expansion.

LOSS OF CONSCIOUSNESS

In loss of consciousness, did the patient "fit and fall" or "fall and fit"? That is, did a neurologic event precipitate the fall or did the fall occur accidentally, with the patient then hitting the head and losing consciousness? Was there associated seizure activity, tongue biting, or urinary incontinence? These are indicative of an epileptic seizure. Other questions about loss of consciousness are similar to those mentioned above for "dizziness".

Following the History Of the Present Illness, a review of the patient's past general medical history may provide important information. A history of hypertension, diabetes, trauma, infection, tumors, allergies, surgery, cardiac, renal, hepatic, neurologic disease, or psychiatric illness may provide clues as to the origin of the neurologic symptoms.

The history of alcohol and other drug intake is particularly important as many drugs have neurologic side effects. The family-social history may reveal relevant hereditary patterns, emotional stresses, or occupational exposure to toxic substances that relate to the problem.

A general physical exam may provide invaluable information, as neurologic symptoms often result from systemic diseases. Specific details of the neurologic component of the exam are presented in the following chapter.

Chapter 3

THE NEUROLOGIC EXAM

Mental status
Cranial nerves
Motor
Sensory
Coordination
Reflexes

MENTAL STATUS

KEY POINT: "FOGS"

1. **F**amily story of memory loss
2. **O**rientation
3. **G**eneral information
4. **S**pelling

In testing mental status during a neurological exam, a critical function one wishes to assess is memory, particularly recent memory. Recent memory tends to disappear before older memories when there is brain damage. Loss of recent memory funtioning is the hallmark of the *"organic mental syndrome"* that occurs with depressed brain function.

A useful term to remember is "FOGS" (as if one were testing how "foggy" one's mental state is):

First note how "foggy" the patient appears. Is he attentive? Or is there *lethargy* (tendancy to drift off from attentiveness unless

25

aroused), *semicoma* (arousal to noxious stimuli but not of sufficient degree to answer questions), or coma (lack of response to noxious stimuli). Then examine the individual components of the word "FOGS":

1. **F**amily story. Information, from a family member, that the patient has lost memory function is often a rapid and sensitive index of memory difficulty. A patient with a very high I.Q. previously may have dropped to a more average level not detectable on objective examination but identifiable on history. A history of memory decline obtained from a family member often will be more useful than a history of such obtained from the patient. The predominantly depressed patient, for instance, may exaggerate a problem of memory loss. The patient with a true dementia, on the other hand, may deny that there is a problem. If, however, the family reports that the patient is acting confused or is forgetful of things of late, this should raise the suspicion that at least a subtle form of organic mental syndrome exists, even if objective testing is normal.

2. **O**rientation—as to precise time (month, day, year). Explain to the patient that you are asking routine questions and are interested in seeing how fast the patient responds. In this way you avoid insulting the patient with an elementary question. Orientation is useful, in that sometimes the patient appears normal superficially but will make the grossest error on this aspect of the exam (for instance, saying it is winter when it is summer, or that the year is 1935). Disorientation in identifying one's self, in the presence of preserved orientation for time and place, indicates a psychiatric disturbance.

3. **G**eneral information. "Who are the president and vice president of the United States?", or "What are some current events?" An "I don't know" may not be significant, as many people are ignorant of the news. An answer of "Roosevelt" however, establishes a gross dysfunction.

4. **S**pelling. Ask the patient to spell the word "WORLD" forwards and backwards. Spelling "WORLD" forwards establishes that the patient can spell. If so, the patient should then be able to spell "WORLD" backwards. If not, this is a sign of organic mental syndrome, the degree of which can be further quantitated by trying a four or three-letter word (e.g, "HAND", "CAT").

If the patient cannot spell, try numbers, as many people who are normally illiterate are still proficient in the use of numbers.

For example:

a. Ask the patient to count backwards from 100 by 3's.

b. Ask the patient to repeat a 7 digit number. Most patients should be able to do this.

Alternatively, ask the patient to recall three objects (e.g., pencil, tie, table) several minutes after the examiner mentions them. The above questions, in a sense, are tests of short term memory functioning. For instance, spelling and calculation assess extremely short term memory: i.e., the ability to concentrate and focus on the immediate task at hand.

CRANIAL NERVES

Cranial Nerve 1 (Olfactory Nerve)

Key point: test each side with a mild agent (e.g., soap or tobacco).

Testing the sense of smell seldom reveals significant pathology of the central nervous system. In fact, an abnormal finding may be confusing, as it may simply result from an obstructed nasal passage or be a normal decline in smell that occurs with aging. It may be helpful, though, to test olfaction if there is suspicion of a frontal lobe lesion (for instance, change in personality; hemiparesis) or unexplained visual loss, as the olfactory pathways run under the frontal lobe near the optic chiasm.

Soap or tobacco are usually readily available for testing olfaction. Ammonia should not be used as it stimulates the intranasal pain endings of the trigeminal nerve (CN5) rather than the olfactory nerve. The nasal septum divides the nasal passages into two, and olfaction should be tested on one side at a time.

Cranial Nerve 2 (Optic Nerve)

Key Points: 1. Test visual acuity (near or far)
2. Test gross visual fields (finger confrontation)
3. Ophthalmoscopic exam

There are two particularly important aspects of vision to test:

A. Central vision, as tested by the Snellen chart (far vision) and/or the Rosenbaum pocket card (near vision). A nurse or other office aide can do this.
B. Peripheral vision, using gross visual fields.

Central Vision. The fovea, which lies in the center of the retina, is responsible for the sharp visual acuity of central vision. If the fovea is damaged, the patient will still be able to get around with peripheral vision, but will have great difficulty in reading. The patient with such a central scotoma usually comes to the doctor's office immediately, as lack of reading skill is a very noticeable deficit. Some patients, however, may not have noticed loss of vision in only one eye, as they never close one eye only. Thus, it is important to test for visual acuity (in one eye at a time), even if the patient does not complain of visual loss. Usually, either the Snellen "far" chart or Rosenbaum "near" chart suffices. For illiterate patients an "E" chart or picture chart will suffice. The patient should wear his far glasses for far, and near glasses (or look through his bifocals) for near.

If one is not searching for a refractive problem but is only interested in determining whether a neurologic lesion is present in the visual pathway, then it suffices to test for *either* near or far vision. Bear in mind, however, that if one *only* uses the Rosenbaum near card, one will *not detect the nearsighted individual who has difficulty with far vision. Moreover, using the Snellen chart alone will not detect the farsighted or presbyopic individual who has headaches, blurry vision and fatigue on near work.* There is an additional advantage to testing both near and far vision: this can frequently distinguish visual loss that is due to a refractive error from that of a lesion (such as a cataract, or retinal or optic nerve damage). I.e., if the patient reports good vision for far and poor vision for near (or vice versa) this implies a refractive error, which will be corrected by a change of glasses. If vision is poor and there is no difference between far and near vision, one must search more carefully for a lesion. The situation is analogous to a camera that gives blurry pictures. If the picture is clear at one distance but not another, there is a focusing (refractive) problem. If pictures are blurry at all distances, there could be an extreme focusing problem, but the origin may well be damaged film (retina) or a cloudy lens (cataract).

Peripheral vision. As for central vision, test one eye at a time. Otherwise, you may miss significant pathology that affects one eye only. Figure 9 demonstrates a rapid visual field exam by gross confrontation, using finger motion, as follows:
A. Ask the patient to cover one eye and to look at your nose. Wiggle, simultaneously, the index fingers of your right and left hands in the superior fields. Ask the patient to point to, or state, the side that moved (the correct response is "both sides").
B. Repeat the same for the lower field.
C. Ask the patient now to cover the other eye. With both of your

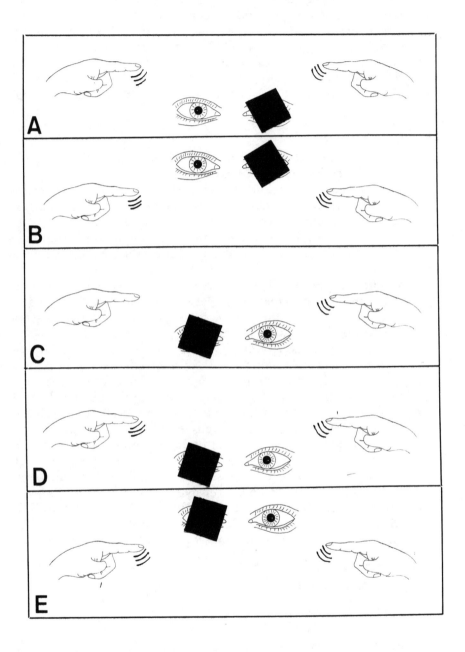

Fig. 9

hands in the superior field, wiggle only your right index finger. The reason to not wiggle both fingers is that some patients, based on their experience with the first eye, may assume that the examiner is now going to wiggle both fingers simultaneously. Ask the patient to point to, or state, the side that moved (the correct response is "the right side").

D. Wiggle both fingers in the superior field. Ask where the motion is.

E. Wiggle both fingers in the inferior field. Ask where the motion is.

You have now tested peripheral vision. The Snellen and/or Rosenbaum charts tested central vision.

If there is the suspicion of a field defect, more subtle testing may be done by the neurologist or ophthalmologist, using a tangent screen or Goldmann perimeter. Your gross motion testing has the advantage of rapidity, not requiring equipment, and usefulness for the patient who has difficulty in maintaining a steady central focus.

Another important aspect of visual testing is the ophthalmoscopic examination. This can be performed either during the general physical exam or the neurologic exam. The ophthalmoscope can often detect the cause of visual loss:

a. The degree of severity of a cataract can be ascertained by the ease with which the fundus can be visualized. As a general rule for cataracts, "If the examiner can see in, the patient can see out". Without the ophthalmoscope, the normal pupil looks black; with a dense cataract, it looks white. When looking through the ophthalmoscope, the normal pupil looks red; it looks black with a cataract.

b. Vitreous hemorrhages, retinal diseases, and optic atrophy can be detected as well as other conditions that relate to the neurologic status, such as papilledema (vision is typically normal in papilledema), and diabetic and hypertensive vascular disease (discussed in further detail in OPHTHALMOLOGY MADE RIDICULOUSLY SIMPLE, by S. Goldberg, MedMaster, 1984). The technique of using the ophthalmoscope is reviewed in the Appendix.

Cranial Nerves 3,4,6

Key tests: 1. Pupillary reaction to light
            2. Lateral and vertical gaze

The term "PERLA" (pupils equal and responsive to light and accommodation) frequently appears on the physical exam report.

Although this is should mean that the examiner tested the normal pupillary constriction to near accommodation, this probably is rarely done routinely—nor is it likely to provide important information. True, a classic finding in tertiary syphilis is that the pupil (an irregular, small pupil) constricts on accommodation, which is normal, but not in response to light. However, tertiary syphilis is rare, and it is certainly unimportant to test the accommodation reaction if the response to light has already been found intact, which is the usual case. It suffices then, to test the response of each pupil to light and move on if that is normal (i.e., PERL).

Pupillary size sometimes is helpful to observe. A 20% difference in diameter between the right and left pupils is generally within the normal range of variability. A large dilated pupil on one side with no other ocular abnormalities is likely to be a benign variant, *Adie's* pupil (unless someone put dilating drops in the eye and didn't tell anyone). In Adie's pupil, the pupil reacts only slowly and slightly to a bright light; there are no other associated deficits of CN3. If the dilated pupil is due to CN3 injury inside or outside the brainstem, it is likely that this will be accompanied by other prominent neurologic symptoms—like diplopia or an altered state of consciousness. Examining pupillary size is particularly important when there is a depressed state of consciousness. A dilated pupil in this setting suggests herniation of the temporal lobe (uncal herniation) against CN3 and the brain stem.

The pupil may be markedly constricted with pontine injuries (pinpoint pupils) and with certain systemically administered drugs (e.g., morphine, meperidine). The pupil may be dilated in anoxia, as well as with certain systemically administered drugs (e.g., atropine, scopolamine).

Testing the pupillary response to light may help to confirm a lesion of CN2 or CN3 (see figure 4).

Lateral and Vertical Gaze. Ask the patient to follow your finger, which you hold vertically and move horizontally, and then hold horizontally and move vertically. Ask how many fingers the patient sees. Also look for nystagmus.

If the patient reports diplopia with a particular finger position, note the position, as it will be useful in determining which eye muscle is involved, and then test one eye at a time; true diplopia should disappear when one eye is occluded, unless there is the rare occurrence of a dislocated lens or a detached retina. (Sometimes a patient says "double vision" but means blurry vision).

Slight nystagmus at extreme lateral positions of gaze is normal.

Confirm this on a normal individual. Marked nystagmus on extreme lateral gaze, or any nystagmus on forward gaze is abnormal. *Jerk nystagmus*, with a fast and slow component, suggests a peripheral or central nervous system lesion. *Vertical nystagmus* suggests a brain stem lesion. *Pendular nystagmus* (equal to and fro excursions) suggests a congenital condition, or blindness since early childhood. Ask the patient with pendular nystagmus whether the condition has always been present.

Cranial Nerve 5 (Trigeminal nerve)

Key test: double simultaneous stimulation, with pin or light touch.

Double simultaneous stimulation of CN5 is most conveniently performed at the time of the general sensory exam of the extremities, and the technique is described in that section, page 35.

A *CNS* lesion that compromises CN5 sensory function most likely will involve all three divisions of CN5, so it is really only necessary to test one point on each cheek on routine exam, to rule out CNS compromise of CN5. If a peripheral nerve lesion of CN5 causes a sensory deficit over one of the three CN5 dermatomes (ophthalmic, maxillary, mandibular), most likely the patient will report this without your having to perform an exam. Thus, testing all three divisions is generally unnecessary unless the patient reports a sensory loss over a particular nerve division or there is some other reason to suspect a nerve division lesion. It is also unnecessary to test the corneal blink reflex (on touching the cornea with a wisp of cotton) unless one already suspects a CN5 or CN7 lesion. The corneal blink reflex depends on CN5 to relay sensation to the brain stem and on CN7 (facial nerve) to cause constriction (bilaterally) of the orbicularis oculi muscles (CN7). This test is useful to confirm a deficit of either CN5 or CN7 in the eye region.

Cranial Nerve 7 (Facial nerve)

Key test: smile

Testing this nerve is a critical part of the neurologic examination. Ask the patient to smile, noting whether there is weakness, on either side, of elevation of the corner of the mouth. Often, weakness is apparent even without this maneuver, as there is noticeable flattening of the nasolabial fold. Lesions of the cerebral cortex or its pathway to the motor nucleus of the facial nerve in the pons will cause contralateral weakness of the mouth—but not the forehead. Thus, the typical cerebral stroke results in weakness in elevating the corner of the mouth but no significant weakness in wrinkling the brow. In Bell's palsy, or other forms of *peripheral* nerve damage to CN7, where the nerve is injured between the pons and face, there is *total* facial paralysis on one side: i.e., weakness of elevating the corner of the mouth as well as closing the eye and wrinkling the brow. Thus, if there is weakness of the mouth, one must test for weakness of brow wrinkling to determine whether the lesion is central or peripheral. On the other hand, if elevation of the corner of the mouth is normal (as is true in the great majority of physical examinations), there is little point in continuing further the examination of CN7, as one is not likely to find a paralysis of the brow and eyelid.

Cranial Nerve 8 (Vestibulocochlear nerve)

Key test: hear fingertips moving

With your hands opposite the ears of the patient, rub together the thumb and index fingers of either your right or left hand. Ask the patient to point to the ear in which he hears the sound. This is a rapid screen for hearing. If there is a defect, determine whether it is a *conductive* defect (e.g., wax in the ear, damaged drum or ossicles) or a *sensorineural* defect. This can be accomplished without tuning forks simply by asking the patient to hum. In conductive defects, the poorly hearing ear hears the hum louder. In sensorineural deficits, the normal ear hears the hum louder. (Try this by sticking a finger in your ear and humming. The ear with the finger in it hears the sound louder.)

Cranial Nerves 9,10 (Glossopharyngeal, Vagus)

Key test: gag reflex

These nerves are tested together by inducing a brief gag reflex. This may be performed when one examines the pharynx and depresses the tongue with a tongue depressor. Touch the soft palate or pharynx. When the gag occurs, note whether or not the soft palate retracts symmetrically. If the nerve injury is one-sided, the palate will retract to the normal side. Compromise of these nerves is extraordinarily rare, and generally this unpleasant test can be omitted.

Cranial Nerve 11 (Accessory nerve)

Key test: Shoulder elevation.

This nerve is rarely damaged except during neck injuries. This simple test generally suffices: Ask the patient to raise his shoulders (trapezius contraction) against the manual resistance of the examiner. One can also test for sternocleidomastoid function by assessing the strength of lateral head rotation against the manual resistance of the examiner, but this is generally unnecessary, unless the result of trapezius testing is abnormal.

Cranial Nerve 12 (Hypoglossal nerve)

Key test: Stick out the tongue

If there is weakness on one side of the tongue, the tongue will deviate to that side. It is rare for this nerve to be affected, but the test is easy to perform.

EXTREMITIES: MOTOR EXAM

Key tests: 1. Drift of upper extremity (and of lower extremity if there is a question of lower extremity weakness)
2. Hand grasp and toe and foot dorsiflexion
3. Testing of other muscles, when their proper function is in question.

If one had all the time in the world, one could try to test every joint in the body for flexion, extension and other movements. By understanding the major aims of the examination, the approach may be shortened. If the examiner wishes to determine whether there has been a lesion to the brain stem or cerebrum that has caused extremity weakness, one of the simplest, most rapid and subtle tests is for drift: Ask the patient to close his eyes and hold his arms horizontally forward, palm up for about 15 — 30 seconds. If there is weakness of the upper extremity, the hand on the affected side will slowly drop or rotate inward (pronate). (While waiting to observe for drift, time may be saved by simultaneously testing something else, such as strength of toe and foot dorsiflexion).

To test lower extremity drift, have the patient lie on his stomach, with knees bent and legs pointing vertically. Within about ½ minute, the leg on the weak side will tend to waver and drop. A common motor pattern in cerebral hemisphere stroke is drift, and flattening of the nasolabial fold on the weak side. Frequently there will also be a homonymous hemianopia of the visual field on the weak side. Weakness of hand grasp and toe and foot dorsiflexion are also commonly seen in upper motor neuron injury. An easy, nonawkward way to test the strength of a hand grasp is for you to cross your hands and ask the patient to grasp your index and middle fingers (try it and you'll see why crossing your hands is less awkward). The patient will grasp your right fingers with his right hand and left fingers with his left hand. Determine the ease with which you can pull your fingers out. Toe and foot dorsiflexion are tested by asking the patient to move the toe and foot against the manual resistance of the examiner.

If you suspect a peripheral injury to nerve or muscle (e.g., the patient presents with local numbness along a dermatome, pain radiating down the extremity, a history of trauma to the neck or extremity, or complaints of weakness of an extremity of uncertain cause), then more formal testing of the extremity is in order. It is most simple to remember to test all the joints for all their kinds of motion. I.e., test flexion and extension of the shoulder, elbow, wrist and fingers; abduction of the shoulder and fingers; opposition of the thumb and small finger, etc. Opposition may be tested by having the patient hold a piece of paper tightly between the thumb and another finger, while the examiner attempts to remove the paper.

The motor exam will be invalid if the patient cannot perform because of pain.

In Parkinson's disease, a stepwise "cogwheel" rigidity may be felt on passive flexion and extension of the joints, particularly the wrist.

EXTREMITIES: SENSORY EXAM

Key tests: 1. Pain sensation—use double simultaneous stimulation
2. Proprioception—test big toe

Pain

It is rarely useful to test all the dermatomes and turn the patient into a pincushion. Generally, if a patient has loss of sensation, or tingling, or burning over a particular dermatome, he will outline the strip-like dermatome area with his own fingers. This will obviate the need for extensive pin testing, except for confirmation in the region outlined by the patient. Cerebral lesions (e.g., stroke, tumor) rarely present as dermatome deficits; therefore, there is more likely to be a general area deficit, such as the whole extremity. When testing for pain sensation in a suspected cerebral lesion, *double simultaneous stimulation* is a very subtle and rapid test, as follows:

Take two pins (safety pins, or #18–20 gauge IV needles) and position them on the dorsum of the patient's hands (his hands are resting on his lap and his eyes are closed). Ask the patient what he feels on each hand—"sharp" or "dull" (this may require a previous demonstraton to the patient as to what is meant by sharp and dull). Bilaterally apply a sharp needle. If the patient consistently reports sharpness on one side only, this suggests a significant sensory deficit on the dull side. If both hands are reported sharp, keep the needles in place and repeat the question 5 or 10 seconds later. If the patient now consistently reports that only one side is sharp, this points to a subtle deficit on the dull side. This sensory *adaptation* is a key to the double simultaneous stimulation test and is a more rapid and subtle way of assessing pain deficit than is testing each hand separately.

Perform a similar maneuver for the cheeks (testing CN5) and the dorsum of the feet.

Proprioception—stereognosis—vibration

Key test: proprioception of big toe

Have the patient close his eyes. Bend the big toe into either a plantarflexed or dorsiflexed position. Ask the patient to state whether the toe is "down" or "up" (this may require a previous demonstration to the patient as to what is meant by down or up). Consistent errors suggest a proprioceptive problem. Be sure to grasp the toe at its sides, as grasping on the posterior and plantar surfaces may induce pressure that inadvertently gives the patient position clues.

Conditions that commonly cause proprioceptive difficulty (e.g., multiple sclerosis, neurosyphilis, pernicious anemia) are likely to affect the lower extremity before the upper extremity. Thus, it generally is unnecessary to test the upper extremities if the lower extremities are normal, unless there are other obvious problems with the upper extremity (e.g., trauma to the neck or upper extremity causing numbness or loss of motor function).

The testing of vibration (preferably with a low pitch C-128 tuning fork applied to the bony part of the wrist and ankle) provides another way of assessing posterior column pathway deficits. Using yourself as a control, ask the patient when the vibration disappears. Generally, though, proprioceptive testing suffices. Elderly people may normally have decreased vibratory sense; finding an absence of vibratory sense can lead to the mistaken impression of a significant neurologic deficit.

Light touch

This typically is spared in unilateral spinal cord lesions (see fig. 1). If pain and proprioception are intact, it is unlikely that light touch will be significantly affected. If there is proprioceptive or pain loss, one should also test for light touch; double simultaneous stimulation (by grazing the skin or hair lightly with a wisp of cotton) provides a sensitive measure.

COORDINATION

Key tests: 1. Finger-to-nose and heel-to-shin
           2. Rapid alternating movements of hand and foot.

The theoretical aim of this aspect of the exam is the testing of cerebellar and basal ganglia function, as these structures play such an important role in coordination. However, vision, proprioception and vestibular sense also play an important role in coordination and must be considered in making an assessment.

Basal ganglia lesions tend to be characterized by unintended movements while at rest. (e.g., resting tremor, athetosis, chorea, hemiballismus). Hence, they are generally detectable simply by observing the resting patient. For instance, in Huntington's chorea, there may be inadvertant squirming movements of the extremities and head. In Parkinson's disease, the tremor is characteristically worse with the extremity at rest, improving with motion, as in reaching for an object.

Cerebellar lesions result in awkwardness of intended movements and are best analyzed by asking the patient to perform specific movements, e.g.:

1. Finger-to-nose and heel-to-shin. Have the patient close his eyes, hold out his hands laterally, and then touch the tip of his nose. Successive repetitions of this movement will help to detect any awkwardness. In heel-to-shin testing, the patient slowly tries to move his heel along the shin from the knee to ankle and back to the knee. Awkwardness of this action should raise the question of a cerebellar pathway lesion (assuming that conscious proprioception is intact and there is no major paresis).

2. Rapid alternating movements. Have the patient repeatedly and rapidly tap his thumb and index fingers against one another. Test right and left hands simultaneously. (Or have the patient place his hands, palms down, on his lap and alternately supinate and pronate rapidly). For the lower extremity, have the patient place his heel on the floor and rapidly tap his foot. Test one foot at a time. Slowness may result from a cerebellar lesion, proprioceptive defect, or paresis.

If there is a problem with balance, *tandem gait* and the *Romberg test* should also be performed:

In tandem gait, the patient should be able to walk placing one foot successively in front of the other, i.e., walk heel-to-toe. The Romberg test is useful to distinguish among the causes of balance difficulty, as follows:

There are three senses which aid in maintaining one's balance: *vision, vestibular sense,* and *proprioception.* These senses feed directly or indirectly into the cerebellum. The patient must have two out of 3 senses intact in order to maintain balance. Thus, closing the eyes normally eliminates one sense, but the other two still function, and the patient will not sway. If proprioception is lacking, the patient will keep his balance with the eyes open but sway with the eyes closed. If the latter occurs, the Romberg test is "positive". A positive Romberg implies a proprioceptive or vestibular malfunction. If the patient sways with or without the eyes open, consider a cerebellar lesion; it is as if none of the sensory inputs can filter through the cerebellum to achieve proper functioning. (The test in that case, semantically, is considered "negative"; the definition of "positive" is swaying when the eyes are closed, but no swaying when the eyes are open). Suspicion of a vestibular deficit can be confirmed by the report of vertigo (sensation that the patient or environment is spinning). Suspicion of a proprioceptive deficit is confirmed by an abnormality in proprioceptive testing. Evidence of a visual deficit is confirmed, of course, by checking visual acuity.

Difficulty in balance may also occur with a blood pressure drop, especially in orthostatic hypotension. In this, the patient tends to complain of dizziness, or lightheadedness (as opposed to vertigo) in an upright position. Orthostatic hypotension is tested by checking the blood pressure in the supine and erect positions. Normally, there should not be a drop greater than 15 points of systolic pressure on arising.

Balance difficulty may also occur with weakness or rigidity of the lower extremities.

REFLEXES

The major relexes are the triceps, biceps, knee jerk, ankle jerk, and Babinski sign. A normal individual may have very active, or absent reflexes bilaterally; *asymmetry* of the reflex responses is generally more significant of pathology. In using the reflex hammer, one will obtain a more reliable reflex if the hammer is held loosely and swung between the fingers, than if it is grasped firmly in the palm.

A positive Babinski reflex is a very important sign that points to an upper motor neuron lesion. In this test, the lateral aspect of the foot is scratched slowly with a pointed object. Normally, the toes respond by plantar flexion. A positive Babinski sign is characterized by abnormal dorsiflexion of the big toe, accompanied by a fanning out of the toes. The test should not be performed in such a stimulating manner as to cause dorsiflexion of the ankle; an upgoing toe in that case could simply be due to ticklishness. An asymmetric response is particularly significant. Abdominal, cremasteric, and jaw jerk flexes generally are not necessary, as other aspects of the history and exam are likely to provide more valuable confirmative information.

Tests for meningeal irritation. The *Kernig* and *Brudzinski* signs are tests for meningeal irritation as occurs in meningitis and subarachnoid hemorrhage. These tests should be performed in patients with unexplained posterior headaches, fever, or altered mental state. In the Brudzinski test the head is flexed by the examiner; the patient with meningeal irritation reports marked pain in the back of the neck, and responds with flexion of the hip and lower extremities. In the Kernig test, the patient reports pain in the lower back when the examiner raises the straightened lower extremity. Such pain on straight leg raising is also found, however, with low back muscle spasm and sciatic nerve irritation, as may occur with a herniated disc.

EVALUATION OF THE UNCONSCIOUS PATIENT

Key points: 1. Handdrop from over head
2. Pupillary size and response to light (PERL)
3. Abnormal eye movements
4. Grimacing, withdrawal from noxious stimulation
5. Babinski reflex

Of course, it is necessary at the outset to establish that pulse and respiration are intact, as cardiopulmonary resuscitation may be required before proceding with the neurologic exam. The history from accompanying relatives or friends also is very important, particularly regarding drug intake, trauma, or metabolic, cardiac or neurologic disease.

An important aim of the neurologic exam is to determine whether any asymmetries exist in neurologic function. If so, this shifts the likely diagnosis away from a metabolic cause and toward that of a structural lesion, as metabolic problems are more likely to affect the body symmetrically.

1. To determine malingering or hysterical loss of consciousness, raise the patient's hand over his head and drop it. If it strikes his face, this suggests a physiologic problem. If it misses, this suggests a non-physiologic cause, as a conscious patient tries to avoid striking himself. Alternately, cold caloric testing can be applied. A 20 cc syringe is filled with cold fountain water and attached to a piece of IV tubing. The tube is inserted into the patient's ear (check first to rule out a perforated drum, as performance of the test may then be damaging). The water is introduced over a 5 to 10 second period. In normal patients, there is nystagmus with the slow component toward the water (fig. 10). In coma, there is no nystagmus and may be no response at all. In intermediate stages (stupor, obtundation), there will be net deviation of the eyes to the cold water, with or without nystagmus.

The number of other neurologic functions that can be tested is limited because of the absense of patient cooperation. The most important tests are:

2. Pupillary size and response to light. Bilateral pinpoint pupils suggest either a drug effect (e.g., morphine, meperidine, heroin, propoxyphene, methadone) or a structural lesion (e.g. pontine hemorrhage). Bilaterally large pupils may also occur with certain drugs (e.g., atropine and other anticholinergics, early and late stages of barbituate intoxication), with diffuse anoxia, or with structural lesions. Asymmetric pupils (greater than 20% difference) should raise the suspicion of a structural lesion. If the asymmetry is that of an Adie's pupil (long history of the asymmetry and no other ocular signs except for a pupil that reacts very slowly to light), this is inconsequential. If it is due to CN3 compromise, this may be life-threatening, as there may be an uncal herniation. If the affected eye also has a ptosis and is down-and-out, this strongly points to a CN3 lesion.

A fixed dilated pupil on one side is a potentially grave sign, and the neurosurgeon must be contacted immediately. There is high risk of brain herniation causing damage to cranial nerve 3 and the brainstem.

The blink reflex that occurs with corneal stimulation tests both cranial nerves 5 and 7. Absence of the reflex suggests brain stem compromise or peripheral nerve injury to cranial nerve 5 or 7, although it may be absent in severe metabolic encephalopathies.

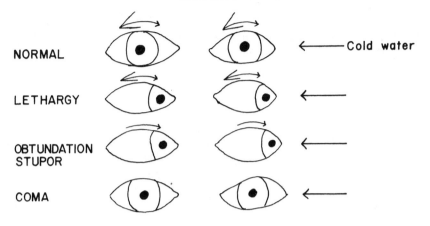

Fig. 10. Cold caloric responses in states of altered consciousness. Small arrow indicates the slow phase of nystagmus. Large arrow indicates the fast phase.

3. Abnormal eye movements. A tendency for the eyes to deviate to one side should raise the suspicion of a cerebral or brain stem lesion. In cerebral lesions the eyes tend to "look toward the lesion", because each hemisphere controls eye movements to the opposite side. The direction of gaze may vary with brain stem lesions. Ocular divergence or roving eye movements, with the eyes moving in asymmetric ways, should raise the suspicion of brain stem depression.

The *Doll's Eye* reflex may be a useful test for brain stem injury. In this test, one turns the patient's head suddenly to one side and observes whether the eyes lag behind. This is similar to a doll's eye which maintains the same position when the head is tilted back. Actually, the response is present to a slight degree in patients who are fully alert, present to a marked degree in lethargy or semicoma, but absent in coma. The reflex is believed to be brain stem mediated, and a total lack of response is believed to reflect significant brain stem dysfunction. Of course, before performing this exam, it is wise to know that the patient does not have a broken neck.

4. Response to noxious stimulus. Twist your knuckle into the patient's sternum, thereby inducing a noxious stimulus. Unless the patient is in deep coma, the patient should attempt to resist by reflex bending of the leg or arm, or grimacing. If these responses are asymmetric, this suggests a structural lesion.

5. The Babinski reflex. An asymmetric Babinski reflex indicates an upper motor lesion. A bilateral Babinski sign in most cases indicates bilateral involvement of the CNS.

Chapter 4

LABORATORY TESTS

X-RAYS

Plain x-rays of the skull and spine are useful in discovering bony defects, such as fractures or tumor erosion. They are severely limited in their ability to distinguish one area of soft tissue from another or to distinguish soft tissue from fluid compartments.

COMPUTERIZED AXIAL TOMOGRAPHY (CAT SCAN)

The CAT scan has revolutionized neurological diagnosis. This form of x-ray can easily differentiate areas of the ventricular system from areas of soft tissue and can deliniate individual neural structures and lesions from surrounding regions. The procedure is even more effective with intravenously injected contrast material that enhances lesions of various kinds. Tumors, hemorrhages, vascular abnormalities, abscesses, and ventricular dilation, which cannot be seen on routine x-ray, can be seen on the CAT scan.

ANGIOGRAPHY

Angiography involves the injection into the arterial system of a contrast material that will outline the vascular system on x-ray. This can reveal whether blood vessels are displaced (as may occur with tumors or hemorrhage), of abnormal pattern (as occurs in certain tumors, arteriovenous malformations, and aneurysms), occluded, or leaking. There is about ½% risk of developing a stroke from an angiogram, but the technique allows visualization of the continuity of cerebral vessels, which is difficult with the CAT scan.

PNEUMOENCEPHALOGRAPHY

In this technique the areas containing cerebrospinal fluid are outlined by air injected into the subarachnoid space or ventricular system. This invasive technique is now only rarely performed, with the advent of the CAT scan.

SPINAL TAP

Fluid is extracted from the lumbar cistern of the spinal canal and subjected to various analyses. At the time of extraction the pressure of the spinal fluid is recorded. A pressure of greater than 200 mm is abnormal. The fluid itself is normally clear. It may contain excessive white cells and bacteria in infection; red cells in subarachnoid hemorrhage, elevated proteins in tumors, hemorrhage, infections, and other conditions, and decreased sugar with bacterial infection. India ink applied to the fluid may outline cryptococcal organisms on microscopic exam. The fluid may also be cultured or submitted for more sophisticated analysis (e.g., immunoelectrophoresis—an elevated gamma globulin may be found in multiple sclerosis and in neurosyphilis).

MYELOGRAPHY

In this technique a liquid contrast material is injected directly into the lumbar subarachnoid space. This serves to outline on x-ray the spinal canal (and higher regions, if the patient is tilted). Abnormalities of the spinal cord, intervertebral discs, or brain stem can be seen. This is an invasive technique, particularly as there is the possibility of inflammatory changes resulting from tissue contact with the contrast material.

ELECTROENCEPHALOGRAPHY (EEG)

Although useful in localizing a lesion to one area or another of the brain, the EEG has largely been supplanted in this regard by the CAT scan. The main use of the EEG is in the diagnosis of epilepsy.

ELECTROMYOGRAPHY (EMG) AND NERVE CONDUCTION VELOCITIES

The EMG involves electrical recording from electrodes that are inserted into individual muscles. Nerve conduction velocities involve the recording of the speed of impulses along peripheral nerves. These techniques are useful in distinguishing diseases that are primarily either muscular or neural in origin.

MAGNETIC RESONANCE IMAGING (MRI)

Magnetic Resonance Imaging (MRI) is a diagnostic technique that examines the interior of the body without x-rays. It detects radiofrequency signals that are emitted by atomic nuclei after placing the patient in a strong magnetic field. This technique is a great advance over the CAT scan in that it allows much greater picture resolution as well as chemical information about the tissue under examination that relates to the tissue's functioning.

RAPID NEURO EXAM

MENTAL STATUS: FOGS (Family story, Orientation, General Information, Spelling). Supplementary: count backwards from 100 by 3's, repeat 7 digit no., recall 3 objects after several minutes.

CRANIAL NERVES: CN1—smell soap or tobacco; CN2—visual acuity (near &/or far); gross visual fields; ophthalmoscopic exam; CNs 3, 4, 6—pupillary light response; lateral and vertical gaze; CN5—double simultaneous stimulation. Supplementary: corneal blink reflex; CN7—smile. Supplementary: brow wrinkling; CN8—hear fingertips moving. Supplementary: lateralize deficit on humming; CNs 9, 10—gag reflex; CN11—shoulder elevation; CN12—stick out tongue.

MOTOR: Drift of upper extremity (and lower extremity, if indicated); hand grasp and toe and foot dorsiflexion. Supplementary: assessment of individual muscles.

SENSORY: double simultaneous stimulation with pin, on hand and feet (check for asymmetric adaptation); proprioception in big toe. Supplementary: determine if dermatomes involved; check light touch, vibration.

COORDINATION: Finger-to-nose and heel-to-shin; rapid alternating movements of hand and foot. Supplementary: Romberg, tandem gait.

REFLEXES: biceps, triceps, knee jerk, ankle jerk, Babinski. Supplementary: Kernig, Brudzinski signs.

COMATOSE PATIENT: Vital signs; handdrop from over head; PERL; abnormal eye movements; grimacing, withdrawal from noxious stimulation; Babinski reflex. Supplementary: cold calorics; blink reflex to corneal touch; doll's eye reflex.

Appendix

The technique of using the direct ophthalmoscope (Fig. 11). Note the two main wheels—one for focusing the lens and one for changing the shape or color of the light beam. The black numbers on the focus wheel represent spherical convex (positive) lenses. These lenses converge light rays. The red numbers are spherical concave (negative) lenses. These lenses diverge light rays. Lenses are necessary because different people have different refractive errors, and the appropriate lens is necessary to focus on the retina. Most of the beam shapes are seldom employed by ophthalmologists, as they are not especially helpful. Most helpful are the large and small circular white beams. The larger round beam is used most frequently and provides the broadest view of the retinal fundus. The smaller white round beam is used when the pupil is small, and there is too much glare from light that backscatters from the iris. Proceed as follows:

1.   Use your right eye to visualize the right eye and your left eye to visualize the left eye. Otherwise a potentially embarassing social situation may develop, and you will need a supply of breath mints. If you have but one good eye, then it is permissible to view the patient head on, although it is still not necessary. The patient could lie down while you examine from a position behind the patient's head.

2.   Have the patient look at a distant object. If the patient instead looks right into your light, all you will ever see is the fovea, which is following and focusing on your light.

3.   Obtain a red reflex (the pupil appears red) in the patient's eye while looking through the ophthalmoscope.

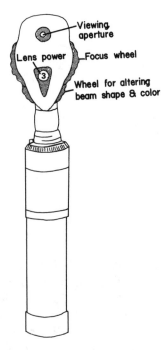

Fig. 11. The direct ophthalmoscope.

4. Move close to the patient, close enough to rest your hand on the patient's cheek. Use the large round white light, unless there is too much glare, in which case the small round white light should be used.

5. Starting with the focusing wheel on 0, move the wheel back and forth until a setting is found with a segment of retinal vessel in focus. The proper etiquette is to use the index finger on the focusing wheel.

6. Follow the retinal vessel back to the optic disc (Fig. 12). Do not be dismayed if your field of view is very narrow, not at all panoramic as in the textbook pictures. No one can see much more than one disc diameter with the visual field of a direct ophthalmoscope. It is necessary to tilt the instrument to different positions to piece together the composite picture of the retinal fundus.

7. The optic disc lies slightly nasal to the center of the retina. Examine the optic disc from *out to in*, first noting the disc margin. Is it well-outlined (normal), or blurred (as in papilledema—Fig. 13)? Then note the color of the disc. Is it normal pink-white, or

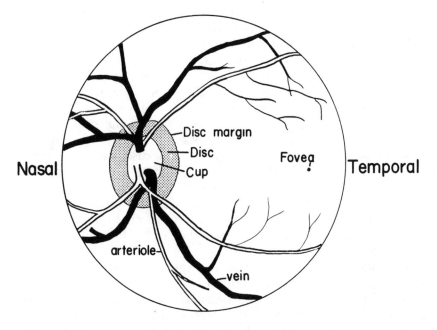

Fig. 12. Schematic view of a normal left retina. Note: The disc margin is well-outlined; disc color (shaded area) is a pinkish-white; the optic cup is a moderate size; four general groupings (arcades) of blood vessels spread to four quadrants of the eye; veins slightly larger than arterioles; no lesions; fovea lies about two disc diameters from the optic disc.

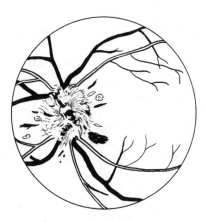

Fig. 13. Papilledema. Absent venous pulsations in cup region; blurred disc margins; elevated disc; vessels tourtuous at the disc level and difficult to follow completely to the region of the optic cup because of overlying edema; hemorrhages and exudates in the disc region; visual acuity unimpaired.

white, as in optic atrophy? Is it angry-looking with dilated, tortuous capillaries and small vessels, as in papilledema? Note the cup size. Is there a normal cup/disc diameter ratio of about ⅓ or is the cup small or large? Actually the cup may normally be small or large, but it is abnormal for it to be large in one eye and small in the other. Normally, cups are about the same size in each eye. Glaucoma causes a large, scooped-out cup, with nasal displacement of the cup vessels. In papilledema, the cup is small or absent.

8.   Examine the major blood vessels that enter the cup. Is there venous pulsation in the region of the disc where the veins enter the cup? You should be able to see venous pulsation in most eyes. If venous pulsation is present, it strongly suggests that there is no papilledema, because venous pulsation is one of the first things to disappear with papilledema. The absence of venous pulsation does not tell you much, since it may be difficult to detect in normals.

9.   Follow out as far as you can (generally just beyond the fovea) the four arcades of blood vessels, each a paired arteriole and vein. There is considerable variation in the patterning. Are there hemorrhages or exudates (which may be found in arteriolar or venous disease or certain blood abnormalities); narrowed tortuous arterioles, as may be found in hypertension and other conditions? Normally the veins have a larger diameter than arterioles in a ratio of about ⅗. Do the arterioles have a normal thin linear light reflex along their courses or is the reflex broadened, as is found in chronic hypertension.? Is the blood column clearly seen in the arterioles or is there copper or silver wiring, a sign of thickening of the arteriolar wall, found in chronic hypertension? Are there retinal lesions?

10.   Examine the fovea, which lies about 2 disc diameters temporal to the optic disc. In young individuals it is seen as a pinpoint light reflection. In older individuals, one may only see a general area of increased pigmentation. Note any *intense* spots of pigmentation, hemorrhage or distortions, within or immediately surrounding the fovea, which may signify macular degeneration. One may also find the fovea by asking the patient to look into the light. This, however, causes increased pupillary constriction, and the excess glare may inhibit visualization.

Dilating drops may be used if it is difficult to visualize the retina. Don't use atropine; it will paralyze accommodation (cause *cycloplegia*) for two weeks. Don't use cyclopentolate (Cyclogyl). It may paralyze accommmodation for 1 day. The latter agents are used in situations where one wants either prolonged pupillary dilation (as in uveitis) or a strong cycloplegia (as in uveitis or in performing a cycloplegic refraction). Rather, use one or two drops of a short-acting dilator like tropicamide (Mydriacil) 0.5–1.0% or phenylephrine (Neosynephrine) 2.5–10%, which last only 6 hrs. These agents require about 20–30 minutes to take effect. Phenylephrine is not quite as good a dilator as mydriacil but has the advantage of not paralyzing accommodation. Do not use dilating drops on neurological patients for whom a change in pupillary diameter may be an important sign. Don't use them in patients with known angle closure glaucoma (they may develop an attack) or in patients who have had an artificial lens implant that clips on to the iris—the lens may then fall into the vitreous chamber.

Glossary

anosmia—lack of the sense of smell.

athetosis—slow, writhing movements of the limbs.

cistern—an expanded area, outside the central nervous system, between pial and arachnoid membranes, containing cerebrospinal fluid.

contiguous—adjacent.

contralateral—on the opposite side of the body.

cremasteric reflex—drawing up of the testicle on scratching the thigh.

cycloplegia—paralysis of accommodative focus.

dermatome—the strip-like projection areas of individual sensory nerve roots.

diplopia—double vision.

dorsiflexion—backward flexion.

dorsum—back.

fundus—the area of retina within view of the direct ophthalmoscope.

glaucoma—a condition in which optic nerve damage results from increased pressure within the eye.

Goldmann perimeter—a refined device for plotting visual field defects, using lights of varying size and brightness.

hemianesthesia—absent sensation on one side of the body.

hemiballismus—sudden flinging movements of a limb.

hemiparalysis—total loss of motor ability on one side of the body.

hemiparesis—partial loss of motor ability on one side of the body.

homonymous hemianopia—loss of vision in each eye on the same side of the visual field (i.e., left or right).

internal capsule—the narrow, funneled area that contains connecting fibers between brain stem and cerebral cortex.

ipsilateral—on the same side of the body.

lesion—an injured focus.

meninges—the membranous coverings of the brain (pia, arachnoid and dural membranes).

migraine—classically, a vascular headache in which an aura (a phase of vasoconstriction, and neurologic symptoms such as nausea, visual defects, and/or motor or sensory disturbances) is followed by a throbbing headache (a phase of vasodilation and vessel edema).

myotonia—a neuromuscular disorder in which, among other things, there is difficulty in releasing a grasp.

nasolabial fold—the skin fold between the nose and either side of the mouth.

nystagmus—oscillating movements of the eyes.

optic chiasm—the crossover point where the optic nerves reach the brain.

orthostatic hypotension—drop in blood pressure in the erect position.

papilledema—swelling of the optic disc.

paralysis—total loss of motor ability.

paresis—partial loss of motor ability.

Parkinson's disease—a disorder of the substantia nigra and basal ganglia in which there is tremor, slowness of movement, and/or stiffness.

pontine—in the pons of the brain stem.

presbyopia—difficulty with near focusing secondary to aging changes in the eye.

radicular—radiating in a strip-like fashion.

scotoma—a focal area of visual loss within a visual field.

subclavian steal—diversion of blood from the brain stem to the upper limb, causing brain stem signs, following occlusion of the subclavian artery.

tangent screen—a black screen designed to test for visual field defects by introducing test objects of various sizes in different positions of the visual field.

transient ischemic attack—a brief period (usually seconds or minutes) of neurologic deficit secondary to transient deficiency in circulation to a given area of the nervous system.

uncal herniation—herniation of the uncal part of the temporal lobe against the brain stem.

uveitis—inflammation inside the eye involving the middle layer of the eye (choroid, ciliary body, and/or iris.

vertigo—a sense of spinning, of either the individual or the environment.

vestibular apparatus—the balance-sensing apparatus within the inner ear.

Index